BREAST CANCER DIET
COOKBOOK FOR BEGINNERS
2024

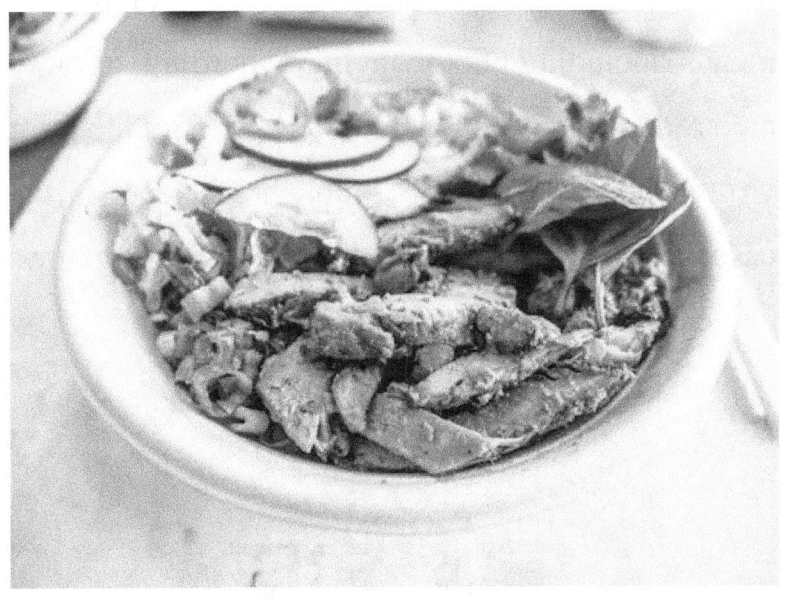

1000 Days of Nutritious Whole-Food Cancer Fighter

Recipes for Treatment and Recovery

Wilbert M. Jensen

CHECK MY OTHER BOOKS HERE

TABLE OF CONTENT

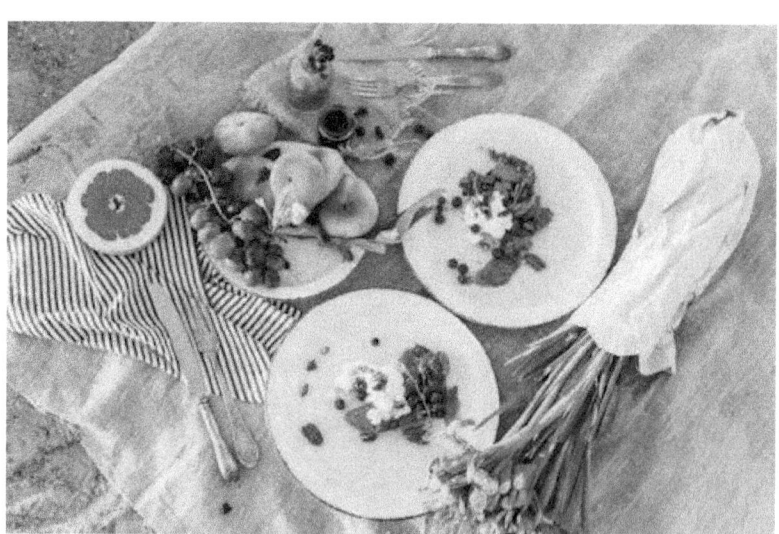

HOW TO USE THIS COOKBOOK

Using the Breast Cancer Diet Cookbook for Beginners is a simple approach that provides individuals with accessible, healthy food customized to their health goals. Here is how to efficiently use the cookbook:

Familiarize yourself. Begin by getting acquainted with the contents of the cookbook. Take some time to read the introduction and any suggestions made by the author. Understand the ideas underlying the recipes and how they might enhance your health, particularly in the context of breast cancer recovery or prevention.

Plan Your Meals: Be proactive in meal planning. Browse the recipes and choose ones that appeal to you and fit your dietary choices and nutritional requirements. Consider making a weekly food plan to ensure your nutrition is varied and balanced.

Gather Ingredients: Review each recipe and make a list of the ingredients required. Before you begin cooking, make sure your kitchen is supplied with the following ingredients. If any items are unknown or unavailable, look for them in your local grocery shop or explore acceptable substitutions.

Follow Instructions: When creating a recipe, carefully follow the directions in the cookbook. Pay attention to the measurements, cooking times, and procedures described. Many recipes in beginner-friendly cookbooks provide step-by-step instructions to help you navigate the cooking process smoothly.

Experiment and Customize: Don't be scared to try new dishes and modify them to fit your tastes or dietary constraints. Feel free to substitute items, tweak spices, or change cooking techniques as necessary. Cooking should be pleasant and creative, so feel free to make each dish your own.

Enjoy and Share: Once your food is ready, take the time to taste it and appreciate the nutrients it contains. Share your culinary masterpieces with loved ones, and encourage them to join you in living a healthy lifestyle. Celebrate your dedication to self-care and wellbeing by preparing tasty and nutritious meals with the Breast Cancer Diet Cookbook for Beginners.

INTRODUCTION

Sophie read the pages of her new Breast Cancer Diet Cookbook for Beginners in a quiet area of her kitchen.

Each dish appeared to offer a hidden promise of vigor and tenacity. Sophie, a recent survivor, had set out on a path to restore her health via wholesome meals.

As she chopped colorful veggies and seasoned with aromatic herbs, she couldn't help but recollect her oncologist's glowing comments for her devotion to a healthy diet.

Sophie felt comfort and empowerment in each meal she made using the cookbook's instructions. The accolades she received was not just for her culinary skills, but also for her tenacity to overcome difficulties. Sophie discovered not just nutrition in the soft sizzle of the pan and the perfume that surrounded her kitchen, but also a celebration of life and the power of self-care in each meal.

DELICIOUS RECIPES FOR BREAST CANCER DIET COOKBOOK FOR BEGINNERS

Grilled Salmon with Lemon Herb Sauce

Salmon fillets

Lemon

Fresh herbs (such as parsley, dill, or thyme)

Olive oil

Salt and pepper

Preparation: Marinate salmon in olive oil, lemon juice, and herbs. Grill until cooked through. Serve with a drizzle of lemon herb sauce.

Quinoa Salad with Roasted Vegetables

Quinoa

Assorted vegetables (such as bell peppers, zucchini, and cherry tomatoes)

Olive oil

Balsamic vinegar

Salt and pepper

Preparation: Cook quinoa according to package instructions. Roast vegetables tossed in olive oil, salt, and pepper until tender. Mix with quinoa and dress with balsamic vinegar.

Chicken and Vegetable Stir-Fry

Chicken breast, sliced

Mixed vegetables (like broccoli, carrots, and bell peppers)

Soy sauce

Garlic

Ginger

Olive oil

Preparation: Stir-fry chicken in olive oil with minced garlic and ginger. Add vegetables and soy sauce. Cook until chicken is cooked through and vegetables are tender.

Spinach and Berry Salad with Balsamic Dressing

Baby spinach

Mixed berries (such as strawberries, blueberries, and raspberries)

Feta cheese

Balsamic vinegar

Olive oil

Preparation: Toss baby spinach with mixed berries and crumbled feta cheese. Drizzle with balsamic vinegar and olive oil.

Sweet Potato and Black Bean Tacos

Sweet potatoes, diced

Black beans

Tortillas

Avocado

Lime

Cilantro

Preparation: Roast sweet potatoes until tender. Heat black beans. Fill tortillas with sweet potatoes, black beans, avocado slices, and a squeeze of lime. Top with chopped cilantro.

Mushroom and Spinach Frittata

Eggs

Mushrooms, sliced

Baby spinach

Onion

Garlic

Parmesan cheese

Preparation: Sauté mushrooms, onions, and garlic until softened. Add baby spinach and cook until wilted. Pour beaten eggs over the vegetables, sprinkle with Parmesan cheese, and bake until set.

Broccoli and Almond Soup

Broccoli florets

Almonds

Onion

Vegetable broth

Coconut milk

Preparation: Sauté onions in olive oil until translucent. Add broccoli, almonds, and vegetable broth. Simmer until broccoli is tender. Blend until smooth, then stir in coconut milk.

Baked Cod with Herbed Quinoa

Cod fillets

Quinoa

Lemon

Fresh herbs (such as parsley and dill)

Olive oil

Preparation: Season cod with olive oil, lemon juice, and chopped herbs. Bake until fish flakes easily. Serve over cooked quinoa.

Roasted Vegetable Medley

Assorted vegetables (such as carrots, cauliflower, and Brussels sprouts)

Olive oil

Garlic powder

Italian seasoning

Preparation: Toss vegetables with olive oil, garlic powder, and Italian seasoning. Roast in the oven until golden brown and tender.

Turkey and Vegetable Skewers

Turkey breast, cubed

Assorted vegetables (like cherry tomatoes, bell peppers, and onions)

Olive oil

Garlic

Lemon juice

Preparation: Thread turkey cubes and vegetables onto skewers. Drizzle with olive oil, minced garlic, and lemon juice. Grill until turkey is cooked through and vegetables are tender.

Quinoa Stuffed Bell Peppers

Bell peppers

Quinoa

Black beans

Corn

Salsa

Cumin

Preparation: Cook quinoa according to package instructions. Mix with black beans, corn, salsa, and cumin. Stuff mixture into halved bell peppers and bake until peppers are tender.

Tomato Basil Soup

Tomatoes

Onion

Garlic

Vegetable broth

Fresh basil

Olive oil

Preparation: Sauté onions and garlic in olive oil until softened. Add chopped tomatoes and vegetable broth. Simmer until tomatoes are cooked. Blend until smooth, then stir in chopped basil.

Lentil Salad with Feta and Mint

Lentils

Feta cheese

Cucumber

Red onion

Fresh mint

Lemon juice

Preparation: Cook lentils according to package instructions. Toss with crumbled feta cheese, diced cucumber, sliced red onion, chopped mint, and lemon juice.

Baked Chicken with Rosemary Potatoes

Chicken thighs

Potatoes, diced

Rosemary

Garlic

Olive oil

Salt and pepper

Preparation: Season chicken thighs with chopped rosemary, minced garlic, olive oil, salt, and pepper. Arrange on a baking sheet with diced potatoes. Bake until chicken is cooked through and potatoes are tender.

Zucchini Noodles with Pesto

Zucchini

Pine nuts

Fresh basil

Parmesan cheese

Garlic

Olive oil

Preparation: Spiralize zucchini into noodles. Blend pine nuts, basil, Parmesan cheese, garlic, and olive oil into a pesto sauce. Toss zucchini noodles with pesto and serve.

Cauliflower Rice Stir-Fry

Cauliflower, riced

Mixed vegetables (such as peas, carrots, and bell peppers)

Soy sauce

Ginger

Scallions

Preparation: Sauté cauliflower rice with mixed vegetables, soy sauce, minced ginger, and sliced scallions until vegetables are tender.

Salmon and Asparagus Foil Packets

Salmon fillets

Asparagus spears

Lemon

Dill

Olive oil

Salt and pepper

Preparation: Place salmon fillets and asparagus spears on foil. Drizzle with olive oil, lemon juice, chopped dill, salt, and pepper. Seal packets and bake until salmon is cooked through.

Chickpea and Spinach Curry

Chickpeas

Spinach

Onion

Garlic

Curry powder

Coconut milk

Preparation: Sauté onions and garlic in olive oil until softened. Add chickpeas, spinach, curry powder, and coconut milk. Simmer until spinach is wilted and flavors are combined.

Turkey and Vegetable Soup

Ground turkey

Carrots

Celery

Onion

Garlic

Vegetable broth

Preparation: Sauté ground turkey, onions, and garlic in olive oil until turkey is browned. Add diced carrots, celery, and vegetable broth. Simmer until vegetables are tender.

Berry Smoothie Bowl

Mixed berries (such as strawberries, blueberries, and raspberries)

Banana

Spinach

Almond milk

Rolled oats

Preparation: Blend mixed berries, banana, spinach, almond milk, and rolled oats until smooth. Pour into a bowl and top with additional berries and granola for crunch. Enjoy!

CONCLUSION

To summarize, the Breast Cancer Diet Cookbook for Beginners is more than simply a recipe book; it is a beacon of hope, a road map to recovery, and a monument to the human spirit's endurance. Individuals dealing with breast cancer discover not only physical nutrition but also spiritual inspiration in its pages.

Each dish is a step toward recovering health, a display of self-love, and a proclamation of resilience in the face of hardship.

As users explore its contents, they learn about the transformational power of nutrition, the healing potential of whole foods, and the profound influence of mindful eating on their health.

Every meal cooked under its leadership transforms lives, lifts spirits, and strengthens communities. The Breast Cancer Diet Cookbook for Beginners is more than simply a cookbook; it's a light of hope, guiding people to a better, healthier future.

Happy cooking!

<u>Contact me here</u>

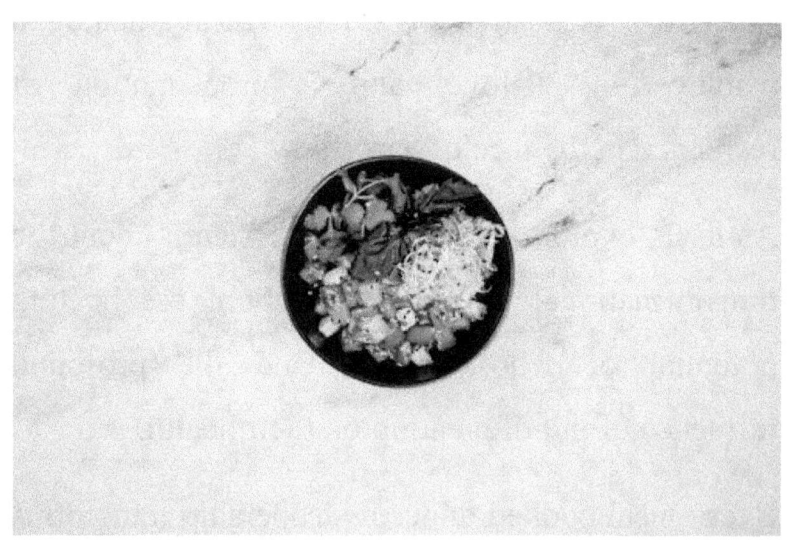